# Mediterranean Diet Cookbook

*Quick, Easy and Healthy Mediterranean Diet Recipes for Everyday Cooking*

**SIMONA SIMMONS**

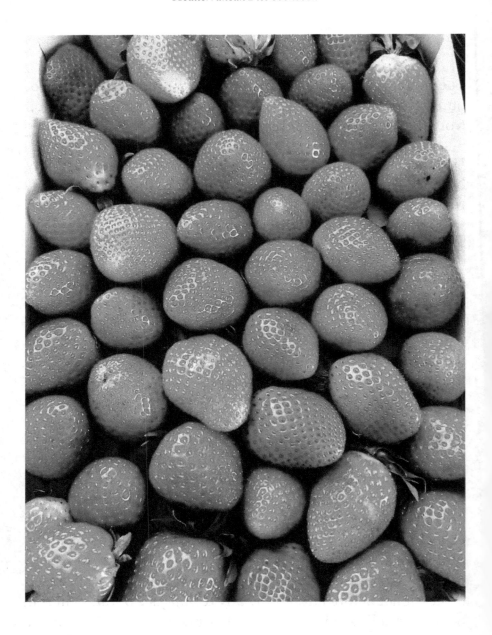

# Table of Contents

INTRODUCTION ...................................................................... 8

CHAPTER 1. WHAT IS THE MEDITERRANEAN DIET?................ 10

CHAPTER 2. HISTORY AND BENEFITS ............................... 12

CHAPTER 3. HOW TO LOSE WEIGHT ................................ 20

CHAPTER 4. FIRST TWO DAYS ....................................... 22

CHAPTER 5. 4-WEEK MEAL PLAN.................................... 24

CHAPTER 6. BREAKFAST ............................................. 28

    1.    CRANBERRY GRANOLA BARS.................................... 28

    2.    SPINACH AND BERRY SMOOTHIE............................... 29

    3.    ZUCCHINI BREAKFAST SALAD .................................. 30

    4.    QUINOA AND SPINACH BREAKFAST SALAD................... 31

    5.    CARROTS BREAKFAST MIX ...................................... 32

CHAPTER 7. LUNCH................................................... 34

    6.    SLOW COOKED COD STEW...................................... 34

    7.    MEDITERRANEAN TUNA STEAKS............................... 36

    8.    HERBED CHICKEN STEW......................................... 37

    9.    PESTO BRAISED ROASTED LEG................................. 38

    10.     PEAR BRAISED PORK .......................................... 39

    11.    SAUCY KIDNEY BEANS WITH KALE ........................... 40

    12.    BLACK-EYED PEA BOWL WITH SCALLIONS.................... 42

CHAPTER 8. DINNER.................................................. 44

    13.    QUICK TOMATO SPAGHETTI.................................... 44

    14.    CHILI OREGANO BAKED CHEESE............................... 45

    15.    CRISPY ITALIAN CHICKEN...................................... 46

16. SEA BASS IN A POCKET.................................................47

17. CHICKEN AND CHORIZO CASSEROLE.................................48

## CHAPTER 9. DIETARY DESSERTS...............................50

18. ORANGE-GLAZED FRUIT AND OUZO WHIPPED CREAM..........50

19. LEMON CURD FILLED ALMOND-LEMON CAKE.....................53

20. GREEK ALMOND ROUNDS SHORTBREAD..........................55

21. TINY ORANGE CARDAMOM COOKIES.............................57

## CHAPTER 10. DESSERTS FOR SPECIAL EVENTS..........60

22. GREEK CHEESECAKE............................................60

23. PHYLLO CUPS..................................................62

24. POACHED CHERRIES............................................65

25. WATERMELON-STRAWBERRY.......................................66

26. MASCARPONE AND RICOTTA STUFFED DATES.....................68

## CHAPTER 11. DAILY SNACKS...................................70

27. TRADITIONAL MEDITERRANEAN HUMMUS.........................70

28. EASY NACHOS..................................................71

29. SALTY ALMONDS...............................................72

30. ZUCCHINI CHIPS..............................................73

31. CHILI CHICKEN WINGS.........................................74

32. RADISH FLATBREAD BITES......................................75

33. ENDIVE BITES................................................76

34. EGGPLANT BITES..............................................77

## CHAPTER 12. EATING OUT......................................78

## CHAPTER 13. RECIPES FOR SPECIAL EVENTS...............80

35. PUMPKIN FLAN................................................80

36. HERB-ROASTED TURKEY.........................................82

37. PISTACHIO OIL DRIZZLED......................................84

**CHAPTER 14. BONUS: RECIPES FOR AIR FRYER** ..........86

38. BACON-WRAPPED STUFFED ZUCCHINI BOATS..........86

39. PARMESAN CHICKEN WINGS..........88

40. BEEF BURGERS..........90

41. BACON WRAPPED AVOCADO..........91

42. BUFFALO CHICKEN MEATBALLS..........92

**CHAPTER 15. BONUS:** ..........94

43. HARVEST PASTA..........94

44. POLLO MEDITERRANEAN..........96

45. PASTA FAGIOLI SOUP..........98

46. PASTA AL MEDITERRANEO..........100

47. TOMATO BASIL PENNE PASTA..........102

48. WHOLE WHEAT PASTA TOSS..........103

49. QUICK MEDITERRANEAN PASTA..........105

50. MONGOLIAN CHICKEN..........106

**CONCLUSION** ..........108

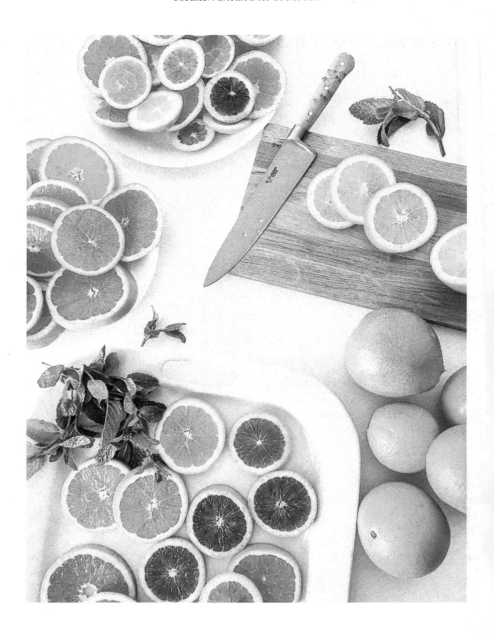

# Introduction

As the name says, the diet belongs to the countries surrounding the Mediterranean Sea, including Greece, Italy, Spain, and France. And after studying the short history of this part of the world, we do realize the vast cultural richness of these states and the diversity of the people and their different lifestyles. One common thing which connects them all is the food they consume and the way it is consumed. Legumes, vegetable, nuts, fish, grains, cereals, fruits, beans, and good fats, these are things which mainly forms the Mediterranean diet. So, it guarantees a good amount of fibers along with all the macronutrients like carbohydrates, proteins, fat, etc.

Since the major focus of the Mediterranean diet is on plant-based products, like grains, seeds, fruits, vegetables, oils, this is probably the true reason that it is full of important nutrients and devoid of fats or bad cholesterol and harmful toxins. From vegetables to grains and fruits, to dairy to meat and seafood, we can experience all using this diet, but it must be in a perfectly balanced proportion. Nutritionists and experts of the field from all around the globe have termed Mediterranean Food as 'The Best Ever," and we cannot deny the fact

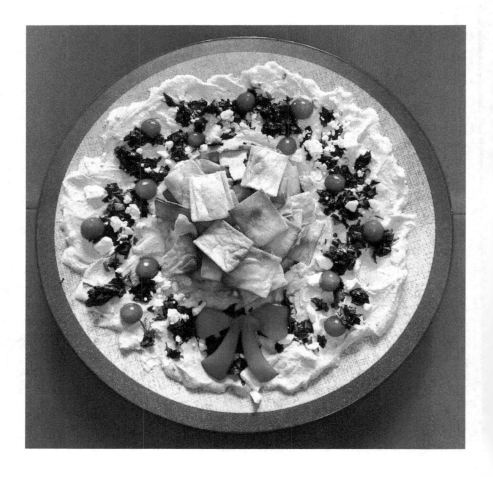

# Chapter 1. What is the Mediterranean diet?

The Mediterranean diet is primarily a heart-healthy eating plan based on the traditional food, drinks, meals, and recipes of the countries surrounding the Mediterranean Sea. To put it simply, the Mediterranean diet is adopting the Mediterranean cuisine and cooking style.

The Mediterranean diet is not a diet per se. You don't really go on a diet. Rather, the "diet" is a lifestyle that has been studied and noted to be as one of the healthiest in the world.

This eating plan or model does not only include healthy food, but it also involves physical activities, eating meals with family and friends, and drinking wine in moderation.

The Mediterranean diet is often also referred to as an eating strategy where you must "eat like a Greek", which stresses the following:

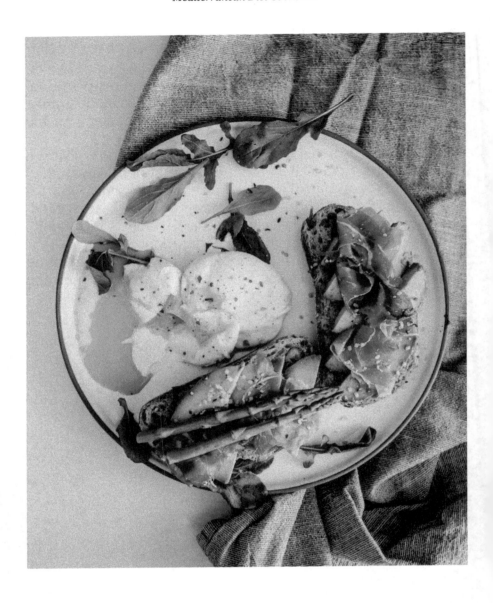

# Chapter 2. History and benefits of Mediterranean food

Origins of the Mediterranean Diet

The true origins of the Mediterranean diet stretch back into ancient times and are lost to history. However, we know that by the time of the ancient civilizations of Greece, Egypt, and Rome, what we now call the Mediterranean diet was commonly consumed in the Mediterranean basin. This diet was like what we have described so far, a diet based on bread, oil, and fish. The ancient Romans were known to consume large amounts of seafood, but as you might expect, the ability to consume fish and meat was closely tied to your social and economic status. As such, rural peoples consumed more bread, fruits, and vegetables relative to the elites who tended to eat large amounts of seafood. The consumption of red wine goes back to these ancient cultures as well. Wine was also consumed regularly by people of lesser means, and so bread, olive oil, and red wine was common in the diets of most people in the ancient Mediterranean world. Vegetables have always played a central role in the diets of Mediterranean people as well.

With the rise of Christianity, bread, olive oil, and red wine became identified with the Christian church, and this helped to preserve the traditional dietary patterns as the world rapidly changed after the fall of the western Roman empire.

Health Benefits of the Mediterranean Diet

We've already touched on the issue of health, noting that in the Mediterranean region, especially when adherence to traditional diets was widespread, the levels of chronic diseases were lower than in the United States, and still are in many cases. This is especially true when it comes to heart disease.

We've already mentioned that a scientist named Alan Keys discovered there was a relationship between cholesterol and heart disease. While we now know that the relationship is far more complicated than he imagined, and unfortunately his research results were misinterpreted to mean that people should follow strict low-fat diets, he also made some important observations about the Mediterranean countries.

- Immediately after the war, Keys noted that people in war-torn areas of Italy and Greece seemed to be in pretty good health. At first, it was thought that obesity was rare because of the war, but it turns out that obesity was rare because of the diet most people were consuming at the time. There was also a documented lack of chronic "western" diseases.

Studies have compared following a high-fat Mediterranean diet with a traditional low-fat diet which is advised after a heart attack. It's been found that the Mediterranean diet rich in fat from seafood, olive oil, and nuts reduces the risk of a second heart attack by up to 70% as compared to following the traditional low-fat diet advocated by the American Heart Association and others.

Studies have also shown that following a Mediterranean diet reduces the risk of a heart attack at a level like that obtained by taking statin drugs.

Regular intake of Fruits and Vegetables lessens the chances of many diseases

We've already noted that fruits and vegetables help supply the body with vital potassium and magnesium. And in the case of leafy green vegetables, they also help supply calcium as well. These minerals help balance out the electrolytes in your body that control blood pressure and heart rhythm and keep muscles healthy as well. If you're getting a lot of muscle cramps, you might want to look at your consumption of potassium and magnesium.

However, the benefits of fruits and vegetables don't end there. Certainly, you're aware that they are packed with vitamins that are needed for health including vitamins A & C that will help you maintain a healthy immune system. Leafy green vegetables also contain vitamin K. There are two types of vitamin K, K1 is important for proper blood clotting, and K2 helps keep your arteries clear of calcium, which promotes heart health.

Fruits and vegetables also provide a large amount of dietary fiber. This helps keep your digestion regular, and it also helps you to maintain a healthy gut biome. Remember that your stomach and intestines are home for a large population of bacteria, most of which exist with us in a symbiotic relationship. These bacteria help digest your food and keeping the right balance of healthy bacteria is important for health. One way to do this is by supplying them with the fibers contained in many fruits and vegetables.

Fruits and vegetables also provide many micronutrients, antioxidants, and so-called phytonutrients which can help reduce the risk of cancer.

In fact, leafy green vegetables play an important role in digestive health related to colon cancer. It's been found that in the absence of leafy greens, consuming red meat can cause the formation of certain cancer-causing substances in the colon that promote colon cancer. Eating red meat alone might cause benign polyps to turn into aggressive cancers. These substances are created by the bacteria in your intestines.

However, if you eat your steak with leafy green vegetables, this doesn't happen. The digestion of the leafy greens keeps the bacteria occupied and the cancer-causing substances they make during the digestion of red meat by itself aren't made. You might file this away in the steak + baked potato = bad and the steak + leafy greens = good files.

Health benefits of whole grains

Whole grain foods, as we've discussed before, provide a healthier way to get carbohydrates. Let's review – if you eat a meal high in sugar, you're going to get a blood sugar spike. The simpler the carbohydrates in the food you eat, the faster they're digested and the higher your blood sugar spike. Blood sugar spikes are bad for you, causing damage throughout the circulatory system.

Whole grain foods minimize blood sugar spikes. Simply put, it takes longer to break them down, so you'll get a longer but shallower and smoother rise in blood sugar. That's far healthier.

Whole grain foods also provide a lot of important vitamins and minerals. For example, whole grain pasta made from wheat berries contains thiamin, niacin, riboflavin, B6, phosphorous, zinc, iron, magnesium, manganese, and potassium. In addition, it's rich in fiber.

To summarize, whole grain bread, pasta, and grains provide vitamins, minerals, and fiber, while providing liberal energy from carbohydrates without the blood sugar spikes.

Health benefits of olive oil
Olive oil might be considered as a magical elixir. While you probably don't want to drink a large glass and should watch it since fat packs a lot of calories in smaller amounts, it's something you want to use liberally, rather than sparingly in your diet.

In fact, olive oil-based diets have been directly compared to low-fat diets in large scientific studies. It's been demonstrated that following a Mediterranean style diet that uses liberal amounts of olive oil reduces the risk of contracting diabetes by 50% when compared to following a low-fat diet. The documented decrease in the risk of diabetes was found to be independent of other factors, like obesity at the beginning of the study or level of physical activity.

Studies in Europe have shown that liberal olive oil use helps reduce the incidence of stroke. In fact, one study found that people who used olive oil daily and in large amounts reduced their risk of stroke by up to 40%. Again, this reduction in risk was found to be independent of other factors like exercise level or body weight.

Olive oil also improves arterial function. As we age, our arteries don't work as well as they used to. They become stiffened and less responsive. Think of them as old pipes. However, researchers have found that olive oil helps to keep the arteries young and supple.

Another area where liberal use of olive oil helps is in preventing or even reversing metabolic syndrome. Remember that metabolic syndrome is characterized by a fat stomach or midsection. Inside the body, people with metabolic syndrome have high blood sugar, high blood sugar, high levels of bad LDL cholesterol and triglycerides, and low HDL or "good" cholesterol. Large studies have shown that liberal use of olive oil can have moderate but significant effects in reducing the waistline, reducing blood pressure, reducing bad cholesterol, reducing triglycerides, and raising HDL cholesterol. This was modest but independent of other factors. In other words, it can help a person overcome metabolic syndrome when used in combination with other lifestyle changes.

Olive oil may also protect against the development of certain cancers. Olive oil contains a phytonutrient named oleocanthal, which helps reduce inflammation in the body. By reducing inflammation, it helps reduce the risk of certain cancers including breast and prostate cancer. Inflammation is also an important factor in the development of heart disease, by the way.

Olive oil contains many fats of all types, including 11% saturated fat. However, it's about 73% monounsaturated fat. Monounsaturated fats have been shown to reduce bad cholesterol and lower triglycerides – so consumption of liberal amounts of monounsaturated fats like olive oil can significantly lessen the chances of a heart attack and stroke. Monounsaturated fats also slightly lower blood pressure. They also reduce insulin resistance (see chapter one), making the body more efficient when processing carbohydrates.

An inflammatory marker that is associated with elevated heart attack risk is called C - reactive protein, or CRP. It's been found that consuming a diet rich in olive oil can reduce CRP by about 15%. And the more olive oil consumed, the more CRP was reduced. By reducing the level of inflammation, you can reduce the chance of sudden death from a heart attack.

Olive oil also supplies some important vitamins – specifically it provides vitamins E and K.

Experts recommend consuming extra-virgin olive oil.

Health benefits of consuming fatty fish

Fatty fish is consumed throughout the Mediterranean region, where sardines, mackerel, tuna, and swordfish are very popular. In addition, people consume many anchovies.

Eating fatty fish has two benefits. By eating fish rather than beef, you're reducing the amount of saturated fat in the diet. Remember that while saturated fat in and of itself isn't necessarily bad, it does raise LDL cholesterol. All else being equal, that's not a good thing (although as we discussed in the previous chapter, the effect can be harmless if your triglycerides are low).

The main benefit of eating fish, however, is that fatty fish supplies the body with omega-3 fatty acids. Omega-3 fats have several health benefits.

•They stabilize heart rhythms.
•They reduce inflammation.
•They reduce triglycerides.

Overall, people who consume fatty fish in large amounts have far lower rates of heart disease and stroke. People expected that they could duplicate these benefits by packaging fish oil in pills, but that hasn't turned out to be as fruitful as people originally hoped. It may be that the omega-3 oils in pills could reduce the incidence of heart disease, but they aren't given in the correct dosages. In any case, eating fatty fish at least twice a week has been conclusively demonstrated significantly lessen the risk of heart disease.

One area where there has been a success with omega-3s in pill form is using prescription strength fish oils to lower triglycerides. It may be that only people with high triglycerides benefit from fish oil and they need it in high doses, but that isn't clear at this time. However, a can of sardines, mackerel or anchovies every day can lower triglycerides just as well as the prescription fish oil capsules.

By lowering inflammation, fish oils may also reduce the risk of certain cancers as well.

It may be the case that consuming the whole fish is important for fighting heart disease, rather than getting the oils in pill form that may leave out some unknown cofactors.

Fatty fish also helps you feel satiated with a meal in a way that lean meat will not. Although salmon isn't consumed in the Mediterranean region, it's a perfectly acceptable food since it has a similar nutrition profile to sardines and mackerel.

Health benefits of nuts and seeds

Nuts and seeds provide many key nutrients that lead to a healthier lifestyle. At the forefront of the many health benefits of nuts is that like olive oil, nuts contain a large amount of healthy monounsaturated fat. Nuts also contain many minerals they are good sources of potassium, magnesium, and some nuts have significant amounts of calcium. If you recall from our discussion about the origins of the DASH diet, nuts have many of the nutrients that are necessary to bring your electrolytes into balance and achieve or maintain healthy blood pressure levels. The monounsaturated fats found in nuts also contribute to health in the same way that olive oil contributes to health, helping to reduce inflammation and improve blood lipids. Nuts are high in calories, so they are restricted on the DASH diet. On a Mediterranean diet, you can eat as many as you like if you don't overeat (eat past being full).

The monounsaturated fats found in nuts help lower bad cholesterol. In fact, studies that examine the consumption of nuts have found that people who eat nuts daily have lower rates of heart attacks and stroke.

Red wine contains many phytonutrients and antioxidants. Moderate consumption of alcohol has even been shown to increase lifespan. This effect is known as the "J-curve". That is, relative to moderate drinkers, those who don't drink at all have an elevated risk of death. While there is a sweet spot where you get the most benefit, drinking beyond that begins to increase your risk of cancer and other problems like stomach ulcers and bleeding. So, people who are heavy drinkers tend to have a much higher risk of death as compared to people who don't drink or moderate drinkers.

Red wine has also been associated with a lower risk of a heart attack. France has low death rates due to heart disease despite high fat consumption, and red wine is believed to be the reason. It might raise HDL cholesterol slightly and thins the blood a little bit that may reduce the risk of blood clots that could cause heart attacks and strokes (when consumed in moderation, heavy drinkers have a serious risk of internal bleeding).

Some studies have also shown that red wine can help maintain healthy levels of omega-3 fats and maintain healthy blood sugar levels.

However, it almost goes without saying – if you don't drink now, you're probably better off not starting. And if you have problems controlling alcohol consumption you probably shouldn't drink at all.

After the fall of the western Roman empire, the Arab world had a large influence on dietary patterns in the Mediterranean basin. This led to an increased prominence of fruit consumption, including citrus fruits like oranges and lemons. Islamic culture also had an influence on the use of spices by Europeans, but this was generally confined to the upper socioeconomic classes. However, it set the stage for the development of the modern idea of the Mediterranean diet.

The voyages of Europeans to the Americas also had a large influence on the development of the Mediterranean diet. This led to the introduction of the tomato and potato into European diets, and the tomato has become associated with the Mediterranean style of eating. This red fruit is extremely nutritious and livens up salads in addition to being well-suited for making tasty sauces.

# Chapter 3. How to Lose Weight by Eating Healthy?

If you are wondering about the initial loss of weight on any diet, it really did happen. It wasn't the handiwork of a faulty scale. There is no doubt that you can lose some weight when you get on any kind of diet. Weight loss is real.

However, it is unsustainable.

When you get on a diet, you restrict the number of calories ingested by you.

This means that if you are running your body on 2500 calories per day, your body gets used to the process. It runs all the metabolic functions in a manner that they consume around these many calories. Yes, it is a fact that your body burns several calories every day.

The number of calories burned by your body in the idle state when you do nothing for a day besides respirating is called the Basal Metabolic Rate or BMR. It is the minimum calorie requirement of your body to carry out all the metabolic functions smoothly. Diets try to bring down the number of calories below the BMR.

For instance, if your BMR is 2000, diets would try to lower your intake to 1500 calories. This means that you would be supplying 500 calories lesser than required and expect your body to fulfill the shortage from the stored fat. This is the next logical thing to do. However, it is not a prudent thing to do, and your body knows better.

It has passed through millions of years of the evolutionary process, and it knows that if it starts depleting its stores at the drop of a hat, there might not be any reserve needed when you really need it to survive in the actual famine periods. Hence, it doesn't start burning the fat deposits. It reduces its energy expenditure and starts rationing in the lavish use of energy.

A large part of the energy in our body is spent on making it feel comfortable. Fending off heat and cold is a part of the process. To provide insulation against heat and cold, our body stores water in large quantity. Keeping that water hot or cold as per the season's requirement consumes a lot of energy. As soon as your body senses substantial energy shortage, it starts dumping excess water. It knows that staying alive for longer is more important than feeling warm or comfy.

This is a reason, people who begin dieting become very sensitive to hot and cold. They have a shaky feeling within. They also become very cranky as the body is actively looking for the restoration of the usual supply of energy.

# Chapter 4. First two days of detoxification from junk food

Detoxification has gained a nasty reputation these past years. While there are countless detox products that claim to be "the only weight loss solution", we all know by now that liquid diets simply don't work on their own. You may experience a sudden drop in your weight in the beginning, but usually that also means a drop-in nutrients and energy. It may help you get a jumpstart in your weight loss journey, but it also gets difficult to sustain along the way. A tea detox, or teat ox as most celebrities like to call it, is a much healthier approach to detoxifying your body. Instead of replacing full meals with a liquid drink, you only need to add a few cups of herbal tea to your already existing, nourishing diet. This means that you can still have all the fruits and vegetables you want even while you're trying to cleanse your body of all the harmful toxins that are trapped in your bloodstream.

Because detox tea is so easy to incorporate into anyone's lifestyle, it's no wonder that countless celebrities now swear by its amazing effects. But what is it about tea that makes it the best weight loss solution on the market today? Here's how tea can help you get started on a healthier and happier way of life.

According to a 2013 study conducted by American researches, going a tea-drinking binge has a wide array of benefits that covers almost every area of the human body. From lowering your risk of stroke, to increasing mental performance, tea is packed with catechins that can help you keep your energy level up even with less calorie consumption. This is probably the main reason why tea drinkers cope better both physically and emotionally when they make changes to their lifestyle.

High quality teas, both green and black, are rich in antioxidants that can help boost the body's natural cleansing ability.

Antioxidants play a crucial role in the detoxification process because it reduces oxidative stress levels significantly and gets rid of free radicals from the body. While drinking tea alone isn't enough to get the job done, it can make the detoxifying process much easier for the body. It's considered to be harmless compared to many detox products that are designed to just mess up the body's natural cycle.

And because there are teas specifically blended with additional ingredients like lemongrass, dandelion, and even milk thistle, you're sure to get more benefits from doing a teat ox than a traditional detox. You can choose the perfect tea blend that will help you meet your specific health and fitness goals. If you're looking for a detoxifying drink that will alleviate stress on the liver, an herbal infusion with ginger for example can clean your bloodstream more efficiently. It's just a matter of finding the right tea blend that will suit not just your mood or taste, but also complement your body system.

# Chapter 5. 4-week meal plan

| DAY | BREAKFAST | MAINS | DESSERTS |
|---|---|---|---|
| 1 | Cranberry Granola Bars | Garlicky Roasted Chicken | Greek Yogurt Frosted Zucchini Cupcakes with |
| 2 | Breakfast Kale Frittata | Tomato Roasted Feta | Apricots and Mascarpone Cream |
| 3 | Homemade Granola Bowl | Feta Stuffed Pork Chops | Minty Orange Greek Yogurt |
| 4 | Mushroom Frittata | Creamy Smoked Salmon Pasta | Apricot Almond Dips |
| 5 | Apple muffins | Roasted Chicken in Salt Crust | Rustic Raspberry and Fig Mini Crostatas |
| 6 | Creamy Millet | Roasted Red Bell Pepper Chicken Stew | Pasta Flora or Greek Tart with Apricot Jam |
| 7 | Rice Pudding | Potato Salmon Casserole | Frozen Strawberry Greek Yogurt |

| 8 | Spiced Morning Omelet | Mediterranean Roasted Lamb and Sweet Potatoes | Orange-Sesame Almond Toiles |
|---|---|---|---|
| 9 | Green Beans and Eggs | Quick Zucchini Stew | Kataifi |
| 10 | Sweet Oatmeal | Chicken Meatballs in Herbed Tomato Sauce | Hazelnut-Orange Olive Oil Cookies |
| 11 | Quinoa Bowl | Chicken Zucchini Ragout | Greek Cheesecake |
| 12 | Morning Egg Sandwiches | Grilled Pesto Salmon | Phyllo Cups |
| 13 | Watermelon Salad | Barley with Perfect Roasted Vegetables | Poached Cherries |
| 14 | Cucumber and Avocado Salad | Couscous Casserole with Peppers and Goat Cheese | Mediterranean Bread Pudding |
| 15 | Spinach and Berry Smoothie | Savory Oatmeal with Mozzarella Cheese | Mediterranean Cheesecake |

| | | | |
|---|---|---|---|
| 16 | Zucchini Breakfast Salad | Rosemary Roasted New Potatoes | Kale Wraps with Apple and Chicken |
| 17 | Simple Basil Tomato Mix | Slow Cooked Cod Stew | Greek Style Nachos |
| 18 | Quinoa and Spinach Breakfast Salad | Mediterranean Tuna Steaks | Lemon Cauliflower Florets |
| 19 | Carrots Breakfast Mix | Herbed Chicken Stew | Italian Style Potato Fries |
| 20 | Zucchini and Sprout Breakfast Mix | Pesto Braised Roasted Leg | Sweet Potato Fries |
| 21 | Breakfast Corn Salad | Pear Braised Pork | Grilled Tempeh Sticks |
| 22 | Italian Breakfast Salad | Saucy Kidney Beans with Kale | Glazed Mediterranean Puffy Fig |
| 23 | Cranberry Granola Bars | Black-Eyed Pea Bowl with Scallions | Mediterranean Stuffed Custard Pancakes |
| 24 | Breakfast Kale Frittata | Vermicelli with Beans and Lemon Crema Fresca | Mascarpone and Ricotta Stuffed Dates |

| 25 | Homemade Granola Bowl | Orzo Pilaf with Herbs | Mediterranean Stuffed Dates |
|---|---|---|---|
| 26 | Mushroom Frittata | Turkish Pilaf with Roasted Chickpeas | Watermelon-Strawberry Rosewater Yogurt Panna Cotta |
| 27 | Apple muffins | Cornbread Squares with Vegetables | Sushi Appetizer |
| 28 | Creamy Millet | Spaghetti all'Olio | Tuna Salad in Lettuce Cups |
| 29 | Rice Pudding | Chicken and Mediterranean Tabbouleh | Rice Burgers |
| 30 | Spiced Morning Omelet | Grilled Tempeh Sticks | Tzatziki |

# Chapter 6. Breakfast

## 1. Cranberry Granola Bars

Preparation time: 2 hours

Cooking time: 0 minutes

Servings: 4

Ingredients:

2 cups walnuts, toasted

1 cup dates, pitted

3 tablespoons water

¾ cup cranberries, dried, no added sugar

2 cups desiccated coconut, unsweetened

Directions:

In your food processor, mix dates with coconut, cranberries, water and walnuts. Pulse well then spread the mix into a lined baking dish. Press well into the dish and keep in the fridge for 2 hours then cut into bars and serve.

Enjoy!

Nutrition: calories 476, fat 40, fiber 9, carbs 33, protein 6

## 2. Spinach and Berry Smoothie

Preparation time: 10 minutes

Cooking time: 0 minutes

Servings: 2

Ingredients:

1 cup blackberries

1 avocado, pitted, peeled and chopped

1 banana, peeled and roughly chopped

1 cup baby spinach

1 tablespoon hemp seeds

1 cup water

½ cup almond milk, unsweetened

Directions:

In your blender, mix the berries with the avocado, banana, spinach, hemp seeds, water and almond milk. Pulse well, divide into 2 glasses and serve for breakfast.

Enjoy!

Nutrition: calories 160, fat 3, fiber 4, carbs 6, protein 3

## 3. Zucchini Breakfast Salad

Preparation time: 10 minutes

Cooking time: 0 minutes

Servings: 4

Ingredients:

2 zucchinis, spiralized

1 cup beets, baked, peeled and grated

½ bunch kale, chopped

2 tablespoons olive oil

For the tahini sauce:

1 tablespoon maple syrup

Juice of 1 lime

¼ inch fresh ginger, grated

1/3 cup sesame seed paste

Directions:

In a salad bowl, mix the zucchinis with the beets, kale and oil. In another small bowl, whisk the maple syrup with lime juice, ginger and sesame paste. Pour the dressing over the salad, toss and serve it for breakfast.

Enjoy!

Nutrition: calories 183, fat 3, fiber 2, carbs 7, protein 9

## 4. Quinoa and Spinach Breakfast Salad

Preparation time: 10 minutes

Cooking time: 0 minutes

Servings: 2

Ingredients:

16 ounces quinoa, cooked

1 handful raisins

1 handful baby spinach leaves

1 tablespoon maple syrup

½ tablespoon lemon juice

4 tablespoons olive oil

1 teaspoon ground cumin

A pinch of sea salt and black pepper

½ teaspoon chili flakes

Directions:

In a bowl, mix the quinoa with the spinach, raisins, cumin, salt and pepper and toss. Add the maple syrup, lemon juice, oil and chili flakes and toss then serve for breakfast.

Enjoy!

Nutrition: calories 170, fat 3, fiber 6, carbs 8, protein 5

## 5. Carrots Breakfast Mix

Preparation time: 10 minutes

Cooking time: 0 minutes

Servings: 4

Ingredients:

1½ tablespoon maple syrup

1 teaspoon olive oil

1 tablespoon chopped walnuts

1 onion, chopped

4 cups shredded carrots

1 tablespoon curry powder

¼ teaspoon ground turmeric

Black pepper to the taste

2 tablespoons sesame seed paste

¼ cup lemon juice

½ cup chopped parsley

Directions:

In a salad bowl, mix the onion with the carrots, turmeric, curry powder, black pepper, lemon juice and parsley. Add the maple syrup, oil, walnuts and sesame seed paste. toss well and serve for breakfast.

Enjoy!

Nutrition: calories 150, fat 3, fiber 2, carbs 6, protein 8

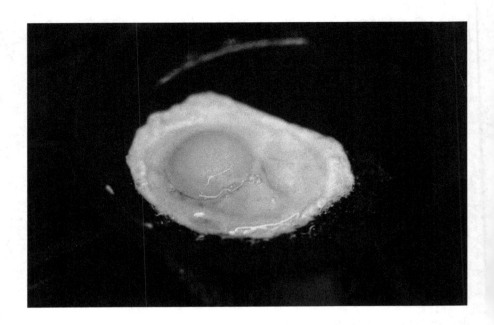

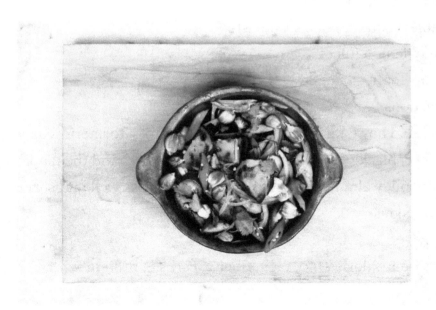

# Chapter 7. Lunch

## 6. Slow Cooked Cod Stew

Preparation time:5 minutes

Cooking time:1 hour

Servings: 8

Ingredients:

3 tablespoons olive oil

1 shallot, chopped

2 garlic cloves, minced

2 carrots, sliced

2 celery stalks, sliced

4 tomatoes, sliced

1 teaspoon Worcestershire sauce

1 cup vegetable stock

Salt and pepper to taste

1 bay leaf

1 thyme sprig

8 cod fillets

Directions:

Heat the oil in a skillet and add the shallot and garlic. Cook for 2 minutes until softened then add the carrots, celery, tomatoes, sauce and stock, as well as salt and pepper.

Add the bay leaf and thyme sprig and bring it to a boil.

Cook for 5 minutes then place the fish on top.

Cover with aluminum foil and cook in the preheated oven at 300F for 40 minutes.

Serve the stew warm and fresh.

Nutrition:Calories:255,Fat:6.9g,Protein:41.9g,Carbohydrates: 4.7g

## 7. Mediterranean Tuna Steaks

Preparation time:5 minutes

Cooking time:20 minutes

Servings: 2

Ingredients:

2 tuna steaks

1 teaspoon dried tarragon

1 teaspoon dried basil

Salt and pepper to taste

2 tablespoons olive oil

Directions:

Season the tuna with salt, pepper, tarragon and basil then drizzle with olive oil.

Heat a grill pan over medium flame then place the tuna steaks on the grill and cook on each side for 2 minutes.

Serve the tuna fresh.

Nutrition: Calories:268, Fat:19.0g, Protein:24.0g, Carbohydrates:0.2g

## 8. Herbed Chicken Stew

Preparation time:5 minutes

Cooking time:1 hour

Servings: 6

Ingredients:

3 tablespoons olive oil

6 chicken legs

2 shallots, chopped

4 garlic cloves, minced

2 tablespoons pesto sauce

½ cup chopped cilantro

½ cup chopped parsley

2 tablespoons lemon juice

4 tablespoons vegetable stock

Salt and pepper to taste

Directions:

Heat the oil in a skillet and place the chicken in the hot oil.

Cook on each side until golden brown then add the shallots, garlic and pesto sauce.

Cook for 2 more minutes then add the rest of the ingredients.

Season with salt and pepper and continue cooking on low heat, covered with a lid, for 30 minutes.

Serve the stew warm and fresh.

Nutrition:Calories:357,Fat:19.6g,

Protein:41.4gCarbohydrates:2.0g

## 9. Pesto Braised Roasted Leg

Preparation time:5 minutes

Cooking time:2 ½ hour

Servings: 8

Ingredients:

3 pounds lamb shoulder

6 garlic cloves

1 cup fresh basil

2 tablespoons pine nuts

¼ cup olive oil

1 lemon, juiced

Salt and pepper to taste

Directions:

Mix the garlic, basil, pine nuts, oil and lemon juice in a blender. Pulse until well mixed.

Spread the mixture over the lamb and season with salt and pepper.

Cover the lamb with aluminum foil and cook in the preheated oven at 300F for 2 hours.

Serve the lamb fresh and warm with your favorite side dish.

Nutrition:Calories:389,Fat:20.3g,Protein:48.3g,

Carbohydrates:1.1g

## 10. Pear Braised Pork

Preparation time:5 minutes

Cooking time:2 ½ hours

Servings: 10

Ingredients:

3 pounds pork shoulder

4 pears, peeled and sliced

2 shallots, sliced

4 garlic cloves, minced

1 bay leaf

1 thyme sprig

½ cup apple cider

Salt and pepper to taste

Directions:

Season the pork with salt and pepper.

Combine the pears, shallots, garlic, bay leaf, thyme and apple cider in a deep-dish baking pan.

Place the pork over the pears then cover the pan with aluminum foil.

Cook in the preheated oven at 330F for 2 hours.

Serve the pork and the sauce fresh.

Nutrition:Calories:455,Fat:29.3g,Protein:32.1g, Carbohydrates:14.9g

## 11. Saucy Kidney Beans with Kale

Preparation Time: 20 minutes

Servings: 5)

Nutrition: 239 Calories; 7.3g Fat; 34.6g Carbs; 12.3g Protein; 9g Sugars; 9.2g Fiber

Ingredients

2 tablespoons olive oil

1/2 teaspoon cumin seeds

1/2 teaspoon Heirloom pepper seeds

1 teaspoon garlic, pressed

1/2 cup shallots, finely chopped

2 vine-ripe tomatoes, pureed

1 tablespoon brown sugar

1/2 teaspoon smoked paprika

Sea salt and ground black pepper, to taste

1 Turkish bay laurel

20 ounces kidney beans, rinsed and drained

10 ounces fresh kale leaves

Directions

Heat a large-sized saucepan over medium-high heat; add the oil and swirl it around the saucepan. Then, sauté the cumin seeds, Heirloom pepper seeds, garlic, and shallots until they are aromatic.

Then, add the tomatoes, brown sugar, paprika, salt, black pepper, and bay laurel to the saucepan; bring to a boil.

Immediately reduce the heat; let it simmer approximately 7 minutes.

Stir in the kidney beans and kale; let it cook, covered, until the kale leaves have turned a vibrant green color. Enjoy!

## 12.    Black-Eyed Pea Bowl with Scallions

Preparation Time: 30 minutes+ chilling time Servings: 6Nutrition: 370 Calories; 11.7g Fat; 50g Carbs; 18.3g Protein; 7.2g Sugars; 19g Fiber

Ingredients

1-pound black-eyed peas

1 bunch of scallions, sliced

2 garlic cloves, pressed

2 tablespoons fresh cilantro, chopped

1/4 cup ripe olives, pitted and chopped

1/2 teaspoon mixed peppercorns, crushed

1 teaspoon chili powder

Sea salt, to taste

1/4 cup extra-virgin olive oil

4 tablespoons red wine vinegar

1/2 cup plain Greek yogurt

Directions

Place the black-eyed peas and 10 cups of water in a large-sized stockpot over medium-high heat; bring to a boil. Immediately reduce the heat to the lowest setting. Cook for 20 to 25 minutes; drain.

Add the other ingredients, except for the Greek yogurt. Toss until everything is well incorporated.

Top with Greek yogurt; serve well-chilled or keep in your refrigerator until ready to serve. Bon appétit!

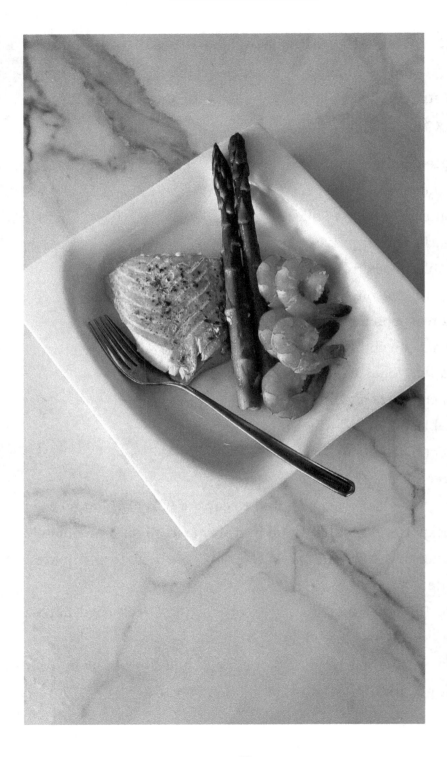

# Chapter 8. Dinner

## 13.   Quick Tomato Spaghetti

Preparation time:5 minutes  Cooking time:15 minutes

Servings: 4

Ingredients:

8 oz. spaghetti

3 tablespoons olive oil

4 garlic cloves, sliced

1 jalapeno, sliced

2 cups cherry tomatoes

Salt and pepper to taste

1 teaspoon balsamic vinegar

½ cup grated Parmesan

Directions:

Heat a large pot of water on medium flame. Add a pinch of salt and bring to a boil then add the pasta.

Cook for 8 minutes or until al dente.

While the pasta cooks, heat the oil in a skillet and add the garlic and jalapeno. Cook for 1 minute then stir in the tomatoes, as well as salt and pepper.

Cook for 5-7 minutes until the tomatoes' skins burst.

Add the vinegar and remove off heat.

Drain the pasta well and mix it with the tomato sauce. Sprinkle with cheese and serve right away. Nutrition: Calories:298, Fat:13.5g, Protein:9.7g, Carbohydrates:36.0g

## 14.   Chili Oregano Baked Cheese

Preparation time:5 minutes

Cooking time:35 minutes

Servings: 4

Ingredients:

8 oz. feta cheese

4 oz. mozzarella, crumbled

1 chili pepper, sliced

1 teaspoon dried oregano

2 tablespoons olive oil

Directions:

Place the feta cheese in a small deep-dish baking pan.

Top with the mozzarella then season with pepper slices and oregano.

Cover the pan with aluminum foil and cook in the preheated oven at 350F for 20 minutes.

Serve the cheese right away.

 Nutrition:Calories:292,Fat:24.2g,Protein:16.2g, Carbohydrates:3.7g

## 15.   Crispy Italian Chicken

Preparation time:5 minutes

Cooking time:40 minutes

Servings: 4

Ingredients:

4 chicken legs

1 teaspoon dried basil

1 teaspoon dried oregano

Salt and pepper to taste

3 tablespoons olive oil

1 tablespoon balsamic vinegar

Directions:

Season the chicken with salt, pepper, basil and oregano.

Heat the oil in a skillet and add the chicken in the hot oil.

Cook on each side for 5 minutes until golden then cover the skillet with a weight – another skillet or a very heavy lid is recommended.

Place over medium heat and cook for 10 minutes on one side then flip the chicken repeatedly, cooking for another 10 minutes until crispy.

Serve the chicken right away.

Nutrition:Calories:262,Fat:13.9g,Protein:32.6g,

Carbohydrates:0.3g

## 16.   Sea Bass in a Pocket

Preparation time:5 minutes  Cooking time:40 minutes

Servings: 4

Ingredients:

4 sea bass fillets

4 garlic cloves, sliced

1 celery stalk, sliced

1 zucchini, sliced

1 cup cherry tomatoes, halved

1 shallot, sliced

1 teaspoon dried oregano

Salt and pepper to taste

Directions:

Mix the garlic, celery, zucchini, tomatoes, shallot and oregano in a bowl. Add salt and pepper to taste.

Take 4 sheets of baking paper and arrange them on your working surface.

Spoon the vegetable mixture in the center of each sheet.

Top with a fish fillet then wrap the paper well so it resembles a pocket.

Place the wrapped fish in a baking tray and cook in the preheated oven at 350F for 15 minutes. Serve the fish warm and fresh.

Nutrition:Calories:149,Fat:2.8g,Protein:25.2g,

Carbohydrates:5.2g

# 17.Chicken and Chorizo Casserole

Preparation time:5 minutes

Cooking time:1 hour

Servings: 6

Ingredients:

6 chicken thighs

4 chorizo links, sliced

2 tablespoons olive oil

1 cup tomato juice

2 tablespoons tomato paste

1 bay leaf

1 teaspoon dried thyme

Salt and pepper to taste

Directions:

Heat the oil in a skillet and add the chicken. Cook on all sides until golden then transfer the chicken in a deep-dish baking pan.

Add the rest of the ingredients and season with salt and pepper.

Cook in the preheated oven at 350F for 25 minutes.

Serve the casserole right away.

Nutrition:     Calories:424,     Fat:27.5g,     Protein:39.1g, Carbohydrates:3.6g

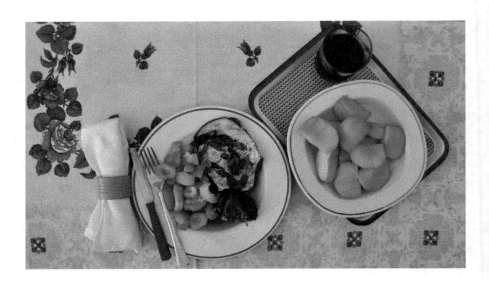

# Chapter 9. Dietary desserts

## 18. Orange-Glazed Fruit and Ouzo Whipped Cream

Servings: 4

Preparation Time: 20 min, plus 30 min chilling

Cooking Time: 10 min

Ingredients:

3 cups fruit (such as tangerine wedges, quartered apricots or plums, or strips of mango)

1 tablespoon olive oil spread/butter divided (I Can't Believe It's Not Butter! ®), melted

Chopped almonds, optional (or pistachios)

For the ouzo whipped cream:

1 teaspoon sugar

1 teaspoon ouzo liqueur (anise-flavored), orange juice, orange liqueur, or several drops of anise extract

1/2 cup whipping cream

For the sauce:

2 tablespoons sugar

2 tablespoons honey

1/4 cup orange juice

Directions:

For the syrup:

Mix the syrup ingredients inside a small-sized saucepan. Bring the mixture to a boil, stirring, until the honey and the sugar are dissolved and reduce the heat. Simmer the mixture, without cover, for 10 minutes and set aside.

For the ouzo whipped cream:

In a medium-sized chilled bowl, beat the ouzo whipped cream ingredients using electric mixer on medium speed until soft peaks form with the tips curled. Cover and refrigerate for about 30 minutes to chill.

For the grilled fruit:

Toss the melted olive oil butter and the fruit in a mixing bowl.

Transfer the fruit into a foil pan (see notes) or grill pan.

If using charcoal grill, put pan with fruits on the uncovered grill rack over medium coals; grill for about 10-12 minutes, stirring occasionally, until the fruits are heated through.

If using gas grill, first, preheat the grill, then reduce to medium heat. Put the grill rack on the grill rack. Cover the grill and grill for about 10-12 minutes, stirring occasionally, until the fruits are heated through.

Divide the fruits between 4 pieces dessert plates and drizzle with the honey syrup. If desired, sprinkle with the almonds. Serve with the ouzo whipped cream.

Notes: I Can't Believe It's Not Butter! ® is a great butter alternative made with oil blends, water, and salt. It's a simple and delicious spread that's all-natural. To make the foil pan, fold a heavy foil into double thickness. Fold the sides up to create a pan and then cut slits in the bottom.

Nutrition: 267 Calories, 15 g total fat (9 g saturated fat, 4 g mono fat, 1 g poly fat), 44 mg sodium, 49 mg Chol., 36 g total carbs., 26 g sugar, 2 g fiber, and 2 g protein.

## 19. Lemon Curd Filled Almond-Lemon Cake

Servings: 8(1 wedge)

Preparation Time: 30 min

Cooking Time: 35 min

Ingredients:

4 large egg yolks

4 large egg whites

2 teaspoons matzo cake meal

2 cups fresh raspberries

1/4 teaspoon of salt

1/4 cup matzo cake meal

1/4 cup blanched almonds, ground

1/2 teaspoon grated lemon rind

1 teaspoon lemon juice, fresh

1 cup sugar

1 cup Lemon Curd

1 1/2 teaspoons water

Cooking spray

Directions:

Preheat the oven to 350F.

Coat a 9-inch spring-form pan with the cooking spray. Dust the pan with the 2 teaspoons of matzo cake meal.

Place the yolks into a large-sized bowl; beat with a mixer at high speed for about 2 minutes. Gradually add the sugar and beat the mixture until pale and thick, about 1 minute. Add the 1/4 cup matzo cake meal, water, lemon rind, lemon juice, and salt; beat until the mixture is just blended. Fold in the almonds.

Place the egg whites into a large-sized bowl. With clean, dry beaters, beat the egg whites using a mixer at high speed until stiff peaks form. Gently stir in 1/4 of the egg whites into the yolk mixture; gently fold in the remaining of the egg whites. Spoon the batter into prepared spring-form pan.

Bake for about 35 minutes at 350F or until the cake is set and brown; remove the pan from the oven, place in a wire rack, and let cool for 10 minutes. Run a knife around the edge of the cake, remove the cake from the pan, place in the wire rack and let cool completely. The cake will sink as it cools.

Spread about 1 cup of lemon curd in the center of the cake. Top with the raspberries. Cut the cake into 8 wedges with a serrated knife. Serve immediately.

Notes: You can prepare the curd 1 or 2 days ahead of time. You can enjoy leftovers on fruit or ice cream. You can also bake the cake earlier in the day and let it cool on a wire rack. 7. Decorate the cake with the curd and the berries just before serving.

Nutrition: 238 Calories, 6.6 g total fat (2.1 g sat. fat, 2.7 g mono fat, 1 g poly fat), 5.9 g protein, 41.4 g total carbs., 2.7 g fiber, 149 mg Chol., 1.1 mg iron, 123 mg sodium, and 36 mg calcium.

## 20. Greek Almond Rounds Shortbread

Servings: 84

Preparation Time: 45 min, plus 1hr chilling

Cooking Time: 12 min

Ingredients:

1 1/2 cups butter, softened

1 cup blanched almonds, lightly toasted and finely ground

1 cup powdered sugar

2 egg yolks

2 tablespoons brandy or orange juice

2 tablespoons rose flower water, (optional)

2 teaspoons vanilla

3 1/2 cups cake flour

Powdered sugar

Directions:

Using an electric mixer, beat the butter on MEDIUM or HIGH speed for about 30 seconds in a large sized bowl. Add the 1 cup powdered sugar; beat until the mixture is light in color and fluffy, occasionally scraping the bowl as needed.

Beat in the yolks, vanilla, and the brandy until combined.

With a wooden spoon, stir in the flour and almonds until well incorporated. Cover and refrigerate for about 1 hour or until chilled and the dough is easy to handle.

Preheat the oven to 325F.

Shape the dough into 1-inch balls. Place the balls 2 inches apart int an ungreased cookie sheet. Dip a glass in the additional powdered sugar and use it to flatten each ball into 1/4-inch thickness, dipping the bottom of the glass every time you flatten a ball into cookies.

Place the cookie sheet into the preheated oven; bake for about 12-14 minutes or until the cookies are set.

When the cookies are baked, transfer them on wire racks. While they are still warm, brush with the rose water, if desired. Sprinkle with more powdered sugar. Let cool completely on the wire racks.

Notes: If using rose water, make sure that you use the edible kind. To store, layer the cookies with waxed paper between each cookie and keep on airtight containers. Close the container tightly and store at room temperature for up to 3 days or freeze for up to 3 months.

Nutrition: 62 Calories, 4 g total fat (2.2 g sat. fat), 14 mg Chol., 24 mg sodium, 15 mg pot., 5.7 g total carbs, 1.5 g sugar, and 0.9 g protein

## 21.  Tiny Orange Cardamom Cookies

Servings: 80 cookies (5 cookies per serving)

Preparation Time: 48 min

Cooking Time: 12 min

Ingredients:

1/2 cup whole-wheat flour

1/2 cup all-purpose flour

1 large egg

1 tablespoon sesame seeds, toasted, optional (salted roasted pistachios, chopped)

1 teaspoon orange zest

1 teaspoon vanilla extract

1/2 cup butter, softened

1/2 cup sugar

1/4 teaspoon ground cardamom

Directions:

Preheat the oven to 375F.

In a medium bowl, blend the orange zest and the sugar thoroughly, and then blend in the cardamom. Add the butter and with a mixer, beat until the mixture is fluffy and light. Beat in the egg and the vanilla into the mixture. With the mixer on low speed, mix in the flours into the mixture.

Line 3 baking sheets with parchment paper. Using a level teaspoon measure, drop batter of the cookie mixture onto the sheets. Top each cookie with a pinch of sesame seeds or nuts, if desired; bake for 1bout 10-12 minutes or until the cookies are brown at the edges and crisp. When baked, transfer the cookies on a cooling rack and let them cool completely.

Nutrition: 113 Calories, 1.4 g protein, 6.5 g total fat (3.8 g sat. fat) 12 g total carbs., 0.3 g fiber, 46 mg sodium, and 29 mg Chol.

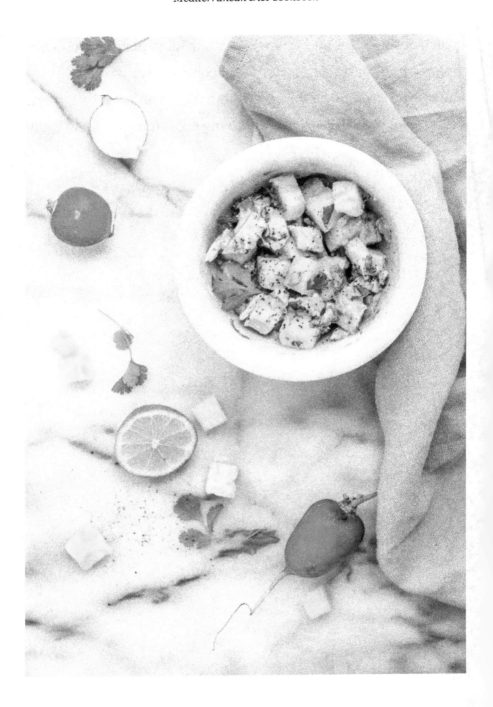

# Chapter 10. Desserts for special events

## 22.    Greek Cheesecake

Servings: 8-10servings

Preparation Time: 1 hr., 20 min

Cooking Time: 30 min

Ingredients:

4 eggs

250 grams whole-wheat digestive cookies

125 grams butter, melted

1/2 teaspoon cinnamon

1/2 cup sugar

1/2 cup honey

1 teaspoon vanilla extract

1 teaspoon lemon zest

1 kilo white mizithra cheese, fresh or anything similar like ricotta

For the topping:

750 grams black cherries, pitted

2 leaves gelatin

300 grams sugar

Directions:

Process the digestive biscuits in a food processor until crumbled. Add the butter and cinnamon, process again until the mixture is like wet sand in texture. Press the mixture into a

## 23.   Phyllo Cups

Servings: 12

Preparation Time: 25 min

Cooking Time: 8 mins

Ingredients:

8 sheets (14x9-inch) frozen phyllo dough, thawed

Nonstick cooking spray

4 teaspoons sugar

For the lemon cheesecake filling:

1 package (8 ounce) cream cheese, softened

3 tablespoons lemon curd

1/3 cup sugar

For the berry-honey filling:

3 ounces cream cheese, softened

1/2 cup whipping cream

1/2 teaspoon vanilla

2 tablespoons honey

Fresh strawberries, sliced (or other berries)

For thee macadamia espresso coconut filling:

1 package (8 ounce) cream cheese, softened

1/3 cup sugar

1/2 cup whipping cream

1 teaspoon espresso powder, instant

1/2 cup toasted coconut

1/4 cup macadamia nuts, finely chopped

Directions:

For the phyllo cups:

Preheat the oven to 350F.

Lightly grease 12 pieces of 2 1/2-inch muffin cups with the cooking spray; set aside.

Lay out 1 phyllo sheet, lightly grease with the cooking spray, sprinkle with some sugar, and then top with another 1 phyllo sheet. Repeat the process until 4 phyllo sheets are stacked, lightly greasing with the cooking spray and sprinkling with the sugar in the process. Repeat the procedure to make 2 stacks of 4-pieces phyllo sheets. Cut each stack lengthwise into halves. Then cut crosswise into thirds; making 12 rectangles.

Press 1 rectangle into each greased muffin cup, pleating the phyllo to form a cup as necessary. Put the muffin cups in the oven and bake for about 8 minutes or until the phyllo cups are golden. When baked, remove the muffin tins from the oven and let cool in the pan for about 5 minutes. Remove the phyllo cups from the muffin tins and let cool completely. Fill each cup with desire filling. They can be filled for up to 1 hour before serving.

For the lemon cheesecake filling:

Put the cream cheese and the sugar into a bowl; beat until the mixture is smooth. Beat in the lemon curd until mixed. Spoon the mixture into phyllo cups. If desired, garnish with lemon peel twists.

For the berry-honey filling:

Put the cream cheese in a bowl; beat until smooth. Beat in the vanilla and the honey. Add in the whipping cream; beat until stiff peaks form. Spoon the mixture into phyllo cups. Top with sliced strawberries or with preferred berry. Drizzle with more honey, if desired.

For thee macadamia espresso coconut filling:

Put the cream cheese, sugar, and the espresso powder in a bowl; beat. Add in the whipping cream until stiff peaks form Stir in the nuts and toasted coconut. Spoon the mixture into phyllo cups. If desired, garnish with additional toasted coconut and nuts.

Nutrition: 161 Calories, 8 g total fat (4 g sat. fat), 22 mg Chol., 148 mg sodium, 20 g total carbs, 1 g fiber, and 3 g protein

## 24.  Poached Cherries

Servings: 5(1/2 cup each)

Preparation Time: 10 min

Cooking Time: 10 min

Ingredients:

1 pound fresh and sweet cherries, rinsed, pitted

3 strips (1x3 inches each) orange zest,

3 strips (1x3 inches each) lemon zest,

2/3 cup sugar

15 peppercorns

1/4 vanilla bean, split but not scraped

1 3/4 cups water

Directions:

In a saucepan, mix the water, citrus zest, sugar, peppercorns, and vanilla bean; bring to a boil, stirring until the sugar is dissolved. Add the cherries; simmer for about 10 minutes until the cherries are soft, but not falling apart. Skim any foam from the surface and let the poached cherries cool. Refrigerate with the poaching liquid. Before serving, strain the cherries.

Nutrition: 170 Calories, 1 g total fat (0 g sat. fat, 0 g mono fat, 0.5 g poly fat), 0 mg Chol., 0 mg sodium, 42 g total carbs., and 2 g fibe

## 25.  **Watermelon-Strawberry**

Servings: 4

Preparation Time: 20 min

Cooking Time: 5 min

Ingredients:

500 g seedless watermelon, peeled, and cut into 5-mm pieces

3 teaspoons rosewater

250 ml honey-flavored yogurt

250 ml (1 cup) thickened cream

2 teaspoons gelatin powder

2 tablespoons caster sugar

10 strawberries, washed, hulled, and cut into 5-mm pieces

1 tablespoon hot water

Honey, to serve

Vegetable oil, to grease

Directions:

Brush 4 pieces of 125 ml or 1/2 cup sprinkle molds with vegetable oil to grease.

Put the yogurt into a large-sized heat-safe bowl.

Place the sugar and the cream into a small-sized saucepan and heat over medium heat; stir until the sugar is heated through and the sugar is dissolved.

Place the hot water into a small-sized heat-safe bowl. Sprinkle the gelatin over the hot water. Place the bowl into a small-sized saucepan. Add enough boiling water to fill the saucepan about

3/4 deep on the side of the bowl. With a fork, whisk the mixture until the gelatin is dissolved.

Add the gelatin mixture and the cream mixture into the yogurt, whisking until well combined. Strain the mixture through a fine sieve over a large-sized jug. Pour the strained mixture into the prepared molds. Cover each mold with a plastic wrap. Refrigerate for at least 6 hours or overnight until set.

In a medium bowl, combine the strawberry, watermelon, and rosewater.

Turn the panna cottas into serving bowl. Spoon the strawberry-watermelon over each panna cotta. Drizzle with honey and serve.

Notes: For a different version, you can omit the rosewater, strawberries, and the honey. Combine the watermelon with 1/3 cup of fresh passion fruit pulp, and spoon over the panna cottas.

Nutrition: 364.96 Calories, 26 g total fat (16 g sat. fat), 75 mg Chol., 69.54 mg sodium, 26 g total carbs., 26 g sugar, 7 g protein, and 1 g fiber.

# 26.   Mascarpone and Ricotta Stuffed Dates

Servings: 5

Preparation Time: 20 min

Cooking Time: 10 min

Ingredients:

125 g fresh ricotta

125 g mascarpone

2 teaspoons finely grated orange rind

30 pieces fresh dates

45 g (1/4 cup) dry roasted hazelnuts, coarsely chopped, for sprinkling

45 g (1/4 cup) icing sugar mixture

For the Frangelico syrup:

80 ml (1/3 cup) Frangelico liqueur

125 ml (1/2 cup) water

215 g (1 cup) caster sugar

Directions:

With an electric beater, beat the mascarpone, icing sugar, ricotta, and orange rind into a large-sized bowl until the mixture is smooth.

With a sharp knife, cut a slit in each date. Remove the stones and discard. Spoon 1 heaped teaspoon of the ricotta mixture into each date.

To make the Frangelico syrup:

Put the water and the sugar into a medium-sized saucepan. Heat over low heat; cook for about 2 to 3 minutes, stirring until the sugar is dissolved. Increase the heat to high and bring the mixture to a boil. Cook for 5 minutes without stirring or until the syrup is slightly thick. Stir the Frangelico liqueur. Remove from saucepan from the heat, set aside for 30 minutes to cool. Put the dates into a serving platter. Pour the Frangelico syrup over the dates. Sprinkle with hazelnuts and then serve.

Nutrition: 115.92 Calories, 3.5 g total fat (1.5 g sat. fat), 26 g total carbs., 20 g sugar, 1.5 g protein, and 1 g fiber.

# Chapter 11. Daily snacks

## 27. Traditional Mediterranean Hummus

Preparation Time: 10 minutes

Cooking time: 45 minutes

Servings:7

Ingredients:

1 cup chickpeas, soaked

6 cups of water

½ cup lemon juice

3 tablespoon olive oil

1 teaspoon salt

1/3 teaspoon harissa

Directions:

Combine chickpeas and water and boil for 45 minutes or until chickpeas are tender.

Then transfer chickpeas in the food processor.

Add 1 cup of chickpeas water and lemon juice.

After this, add salt and harissa.

Blend the hummus until it is smooth and fluffy.

Add olive oil and pulse it for 10 seconds more.

Transfer the cooked hummus in the bowl and store it in the fridge up to 2 days.

Nutrition: calories 160, fat 7.9, fiber 5. carbs 17.8, protein 5.7

## 28.    Easy Nachos

Preparation Time: 10 minutes

Cooking time: 10 minutes

Servings:7

Ingredients:

1 cup nachos

1/3 cup Monterey Jack cheese, shredded

2 oz black olives, sliced

2 tomatoes, chopped

Directions:

Crash the nachos gently and arrange them in the casserole mold in one layer.

Make the layer of black olives and tomatoes over the nachos. Flatten the ingredients with the help of spatula if needed.

Then make the layer of cheese and cover casserole mold with foil. Secure the edges.

Bake the nachos for 10 minutes at 365F.

Then remove the foil from the mold and serve nachos in the casserole mold.

Nutrition: calories 133, fat 8, fiber 2.3, carbs 10.6, protein 5.4

## 29.  Salty Almonds

Preparation Time: 1 hour 10 minutes

Cooking time: 15 minutes

Servings:5

Ingredients:

1 cup almonds

3 tablespoons salt

2 cups of water

Directions:

Bring water to boil.

After this, add 2 tablespoons of salt in water and stir it.

When salt is dissolved, add almonds and let them soak for at least 1 hour.

Meanwhile, line the tray with baking paper and preheat oven to 350F.

Dry the soaked almonds with a paper towel well and arrange them in one layer in the tray.

Sprinkle buts with remaining salt.

Bake the snack for 15 minutes. Mix it from time to time with the help of the spatula or spoon.

Nutrition: calories 110, fat 9.5, fiber 2.4, carbs 4.1, protein 4

## 30. Zucchini Chips

Preparation Time: 15 minutes

Cooking time: 20 minutes

Servings:4

Ingredients:

1 zucchini

2 oz Parmesan, grated

½ teaspoon paprika

1 teaspoon olive oil

Directions:

Trim zucchini and slice it into the chips with the help of the vegetable slices.

Then mix up together Parmesan and paprika.

Sprinkle the zucchini chips with olive oil.

After this, dip every zucchini slice in the cheese mixture.

Place the zucchini chips in the lined baking tray and bake for 20 minutes at 375F.

Flip the zucchini sliced onto another side after 10 minutes of cooking.

Chill the cooked chips well.

Nutrition: calories 64, fat 4.3, fiber 0.6, carbs 2.3, protein 5.2

## 31.    Chili Chicken Wings

Preparation Time: 10 minutes

Cooking time: 20 minutes

Servings:3

Ingredients:

3 chicken wings, boneless

1 teaspoon chili pepper, minced

1tablespoon olive oil

1 teaspoon minced garlic

2 tablespoons balsamic vinegar

½ teaspoon salt

Directions:

 Make the chicken sauce: whisk together minced chili pepper, olive oil, minced garlic, balsamic vinegar, and salt.

 Preheat the oven to 360F.

 Line the baking tray with parchment.

 Rub the chicken wings with chicken sauce generously and transfer in the tray.

 Bake the poultry for 20 minutes. Flip them onto another side after 10 minutes of cooking.

Nutrition: calories 138, fat 11, fiber 0.2, carbs 3.8, protein 5.9

## 32.    Radish Flatbread Bites

Preparation Time: 10 minutes

Cooking time: 10 minutes

Servings:8

Ingredients:

2 tablespoons butter

1/3 cup milk

1 ½ cup wheat flour, whole grain

1 teaspoon salt

1 teaspoon avocado oil

1 cup radish

1 tablespoon cream cheese

Directions:

Melt butter and combine it together with milk. Stir the liquid.

Then mix up together flour with butter mixture.

Knead the soft and non-sticky dough.

Cut the dough into 8 pieces.

Roll up every dough piece into the circle (flatbread).

Pour avocado oil in the skillet.

Roast the flatbreads for 1 minute from each side over the medium heat.

After this, slice the radish and mix it up with cream cheese and salt.

Top cooked flatbreads with radish.

Nutrition: calories 123, fat 3.8, fiber 0.9, carbs 18.9, protein 3

## 33. Endive Bites

Preparation Time: 10 minutes

Cooking time: 0 minutes

Servings:10

Ingredients:

6 oz endive

2 pears, chopped

4 oz Blue cheese, crumbled

1 teaspoon olive oil

1 teaspoon lemon juice

¾ teaspoon ground cinnamon

Directions:

 Separate endive into the spears (10 spears).

 In the bowl combine chopped pears, olive oil, lemon juice, ground cinnamon, and Blue cheese.

 Fill the endive spears with cheese mixture.

Nutrition: calories 72, fat 3.8, fiber 1.9, carbs 7.4, protein 2.8

## 34.  Eggplant Bites

Preparation Time: 15 minutes

Cooking time: 30 minutes

Servings:8

Ingredients:

2 eggs, beaten

3 oz Parmesan, grated

1 tablespoon coconut flakes

½ teaspoon ground paprika

1 teaspoon salt

2 eggplants, trimmed

Directions:

Slice the eggplants into the thin circles. Use the vegetable slicer for this step.

After this, sprinkle the vegetables with salt and mix up. Leave them for 5-10 minutes.

Then drain eggplant juice and sprinkle them with ground paprika.

Mix up together coconut flakes and Parmesan.

Dip every eggplant circle in the egg and then coat in Parmesan mixture.

Line the baking tray with parchment and place eggplants on it.

Bake the vegetables for 30 minutes at 360F. Flip the eggplants into another side after 12 minutes of cooking.

Nutrition: calories 87, fat 3.9, fiber 5, carbs 8.7, protein 6.2

# Chapter 12. Eating out

Just because you enjoy eating at restaurants, does not mean you have to ditch the diet. The Mediterranean way of eating positively encourages making meals a social event. It can be a time to get together and unwind. Their way of life might be slower, but there is no reason why you cannot incorporate it into your own new lifestyle. Here are a few tips to help you when eating out:

•       As you take a seat, have a glass of water. Studies have shown that drinking 17ounces of water prior to a meal, gives you 44% chance not to overeat, therefore assists in weight loss.

•       Avoid breadbaskets. Eat whole-wheat bread at best but save that for home and in moderation.

•       Avoid fried foods, unless you are confident, they are cooked in olive oil. The only to find is to ask, if you're bold enough.

•       Skip the appetizer or share one at the very least.

•       For your main course, chose chicken, or lean pork if you prefer a meat dish.  Or consider having fish instead. Better yet, have a vegetarian plate

•       Avoid dishes with sauces. Chances are, they have ample sugar and salt to make them palatable. Again, you could ask, but if you are at a chain restaurant, they may not even know the answer as it comes ready made in bulk. That's not a nice reflection!

- Choose plenty of vegetables, even order more as a side dish.
- Avoid salad dressings.
- Fruit for dessert is always better. If you can't resist a pudding; share it with a few friends, this way you only have a couple of spoons.
- Enjoy one glass of red wine, and then drink water for the rest of the meal.
- Chew slowly until all the food is masticated, and easy to swallow.
- Think about the flavors of your food as you chew. Simply said, don't just eat by design- discover the flavors within.
- Sit down and enjoy the food. Appreciate what you taste and consume
- Restaurant portions may be large, so get into the habit of leaving some food on your plate.

# Chapter 13. Recipes for special events

### 35. Pumpkin Flan

Servings: 12

Preparation Time: 30 min, plus 3 hr. chilling

Cooking Time: 20 min

Ingredients:

1 can (15-ounce) pumpkin purée

1 3/4 cups sugar, divided

1 cardamom pod, cracked

1 cup milk

1 teaspoon orange zest

1 teaspoon vanilla extract

2 1/3 cups heavy cream, divided

2 cinnamon sticks

3 whole star anise

5 whole cloves

6 large-sized egg yolks

6 large-sized eggs

1/4 cup water

Directions:

In a large-sized heat-safe bowl, whisk the eggs, the egg yolks, 3/4 cup of the sugar, and the orange zest. Pour the milk, 2 cups of the heavy cream, star anise, cloves, cardamom pod, and cinnamon sticks into a large-sized saucepan; bring to a simmer over medium flame or heat. When simmering, slowly whisk in the egg mixture. Let the mixture steep for 30 minutes. Strain into a heatproof container. Whisk in the pumpkin puree and the vanilla extract. Refrigerate and chill for 3 hours.

In a heavy, small-sized saucepan, stir 1/4 cup water and the remaining 1 cup sugar. Heat over low flame or heat until the sugar is dissolved. Increase the heat and without stirring, bring the syrup to a boil until the deep amber in color, brushing down the sides of the pan with a wet pastry brush occasionally swirling the pan, about 10 minutes. Stir in the remaining 1/3 cup of the heavy cream. The caramel will vigorously bubble.

Divide the caramel mixture between 12 ramekins; refrigerate to chill until set. Divide the custard between the 12 ramekins, pouring over the set caramel. Place the ramekins into a large-sized, oven-safe pan. Carefully pour hot water into the pan, filling until the hot water is halfway up the ramekin sides. Cover the pan with foil.

Bake for about 20 to 25 minutes or until the center of the custard is set. Remove from the oven; remove the foil cover, let cool until warm enough to handle. Refrigerate the flans to chill until cold. When ready to serve, invert the ramekins into plates to dislodge the flans.

Nutrition: 338.3Calories, 20.4 g total fat (11.2 g sat. fat), 60.1 mg sodium, 242.3 mg Chol., 33.8 g total carbs., 0.5 g fiber, 31.1 g sugar, and 6.2 g protein

# 36.   Herb-Roasted Turkey

Servings: 8 to 10

Preparation Time: 20 min

Cooking Time: 2 3/4 hr.

Ingredients:

1-piece (12-14 pounds) turkey, neck and giblets removed, at room temperature for 1 hour

1 1/12 tablespoons freshly ground black pepper

1 lemon, quartered

1 onion, medium-sized, quartered

1 orange, quartered

1 tablespoon fresh rosemary, minced

1 tablespoon fresh sage leaves, minced

1 tablespoon fresh thyme leaves, minced

1 tablespoon lemon zest, finely grated

3 tablespoons kosher salt

6 tablespoons (3/4 stick) unsalted butter, at room temperature

Directions:

Preheat the oven to450F. Place a rack inside a large-sized roasting pan.

With paper towels, pat the turkey dry. Rub the inside and the outside of the turkey with salt and pepper. Put the turkey on the rack in the pan.

In a small-sized bowl, mix the butter, rosemary, lemon zest, thyme, and sage with a fork. Rub the herb mixture on the outside and the inside cavity of the turkey.

Put the lemon quarters, orange quarters, and the onion inside the turkey cavity. Tuck the tips of the wings under the turkey to prevent them from burning during roasting.

Pour 4 cups of water into the roasting pan; place into the oven and roast uncovered for about 30 minutes. After 30 minutes, reduce the oven temperature to 325F. Baste the turkey with the juices in the pan. If needed, add more water into the roasting pan to maintain at least 1/4-inch of liquid in the bottom of the roasting pan. Continue roasting the turkey for a total of 2 3/4 hours, basting every 30 minutes and tenting the turkey with foil if the skin is turning too dark. The turkey is roasted when an instant-read thermometer reads 165F when inserted in the thickest part of the thigh without touching the bone and the juices run clear when the thermometer is removed.

When cooked, transfer the turkey into a serving platter. Tent the bird with foil; let rest for 1 hour before carving.

Nutrition: 640 Calories, 10 g total fat (6 g sat. fat), 1170 mg sodium, 360 mg Chol., 4 g total carbs., 1 g fiber, 2 g sugar, and 123 g protein.

## 37. Pistachio Oil Drizzled

Servings: 12

Preparation Time: 15 min, plus 30 min softening

Cooking Time: 15 min

Ingredients:

6 dried figs

2 tablespoons sugar

2 tablespoons pistachios, toasted and shelled

12 slices ciabatta bread

1/4 cup extra-virgin olive oil

1/2 cup red wine vinegar

1/4 cup water

Robiola cheese, at room temperature

Directions:

In a saucepan, combine the sugar, red wine vinegar, dried figs, and water; bring the mixture to a simmer. When simmering, remove from the heat; let sit for about 30 minutes or until the figs are soft. When the figs are soft, cut the figs into halves in a lengthwise manner. Alternatively, you can use 6 pieces fresh figs halve d lengthwise.

Crush the pistachios into fine pieces and then combine with the olive oil.

Grill the slices of ciabatta bread.

Spread the cheese over the warm toasted bread slices. Top with each with a fig half and then drizzle with the pistachio oil.

Nutrition: 132.8 Calories, 5.8 g total fat (1 g sat. fat), 120.7 mg sodium, 1.2 mg Chol., 18.44 g total carbs., 1 g fiber, 4.7 g sugar, and 2.8 g protein.

# Chapter 14. Bonus

## 38. Bacon-Wrapped Stuffed Zucchini Boats

Cooking Time: 15 minutes

Servings: 4

Ingredients:

½ a teaspoon of fresh ground black pepper

1 teaspoon sea salt

5-ounces cream cheese

8-mushrooms, finely chopped

1 tablespoon Italian parsley, chopped

1 tablespoon finely chopped dill

3 garlic cloves, peeled, pressed

1 sweet red pepper, finely chopped

2 large zucchinis

12 bacon strips

1 medium onion, chopped

Directions:

Preheat your air fryer to 350°Fahrenheit. Trim the ends off zucchini. Cut zucchini in half lengthwise. Scoop out pulp, leaving ¼-inch thick shells. Stir pulp in mixing bowl. Add onion, garlic, herbs, pepper, cream cheese, salt, and pepper. Mix well to combine. Fill individual shells with the same amount of stuffing. Wrap three bacon strips around each zucchini boat such that the ends end up underneath. Place them directly on the air fryer rack and bake turning the temperature up to 375°Fahrenheit for 15-minutes. Remove and serve immediately.

Nutrition: Calories: 282, Total Fat: 9.1g, Carbs: 6.3g, Protein: 24.2g

# 39.   Parmesan Chicken Wings

Cooking Time: 22 minutes

Servings:  4

Ingredients:

2 lbs. chicken wings

2 tablespoons olive oil

1 teaspoon sea salt

1 teaspoon black pepper

3 tablespoons butter

3 tablespoons olive oil

3 garlic cloves, minced

4 tablespoons parmesan cheese

1/8 teaspoon smoked paprika

¼ teaspoon red pepper flakes

Salt and pepper to taste

Directions:

Add chicken to a bowl and pat the chicken dry.  Drizzle with 2 tablespoons of olive oil, 1 teaspoon of sea salt, and 1 teaspoon black pepper.  Gently toss to coat chicken.  Place chicken wings into air fryer directly on the rack.  Bake at 400°Fahrenheit for 20-minutes, flipping wings half-way through cook time.  In a pan over medium heat add butter and 3 tablespoons olive oil and melt the butter down, for about 3-minutes.  Add 2 tablespoons of parmesan cheese, smoked paprika, red pepper flakes, salt and pepper to taste.  Cook sauce for about 2-minutes.  Remove the wings from air fryer and place in large bowl. Pour the garlic parmesan sauce over the wings toss to coat. Serve wings topped with additional a2 tablespoons of parmesan cheese.

Nutrition: Calories: 324, Total Fat: 12.3g, Carbs: 9.3g, Protein: 39.3g

## 40.   Beef Burgers

Cooking Time: 10 minutes

Servings: 4

Ingredients:

1 lb. ground beef

1 teaspoon parsley, dried

½ teaspoon oregano, dried

½ teaspoon ground black pepper

½ teaspoon salt

½ teaspoon onion powder

½ teaspoon garlic powder

1 tablespoon Worcestershire sauce

Olive oil cooking spray

Directions:

In a mixing bowl, mix the seasonings. Add the seasoning to beef in a bowl. Mix well to combine. Divide the beef into four patties, put an indent in the middle of patties with your thumb to prevent patties from bunching up in the middle. Place burgers into air fryer and spray the tops of them with olive oil. Cook for 10-minutes at 400°Fahrenheit, no need to flip patties. Serve on a bun with a side dish of your choice.

Nutrition: Calories: 312, Total Fat: 11.3g, Carbs: 7.2g, Protein: 39.2g

## 41.  Bacon Wrapped Avocado

Cooking Time: 10 minutes

Servings:  2

Ingredients:

2 avocados, fresh and firm

Chili powder

Ground cumin

4 thick slices of hickory smoked bacon

Directions:

Slice the avocados into wedges and peel off the skin. Stretch the bacon strips this will help to elongate them. Slice avocados in half. Next, take half a bacon strip and wrap one around each avocado wedge and tuck the ends under the bottom. Sprinkle wedges with chili powder and cumin. Bake the bacon wrapped avocado wedges in air fryer at 400°Fahrenheit for 10-minutes. Serve with your favorite salad!

Nutrition: Calories:  276, Total Fat:  7.3g, Carbs:  6.3g, Protein:  21g

## 42.　Buffalo Chicken Meatballs

Cooking Time: 20 minutes

Servings:  4

Ingredients:

1 lb. ground chicken

1 egg, beaten

1 celery stalk, trimmed and finely diced

1 cup buffalo wing sauce

1 teaspoon black pepper

1 teaspoon pink sea salt

1 teaspoon garlic powder

1 teaspoon onion powder

1 tablespoon mayonnaise

1 tablespoon almond flour

2 sprigs of green onion, finely chopped

Directions:

Place the baking pan in air fryer and spray with olive oil.  In a bowl, combine all ingredients, except buffalo sauce.  Mix well.  Use your hands to form 2-inch balls.  Place the meatballs in air fryer and bake at 350°Fahrenheit for 15-minutes.  Remove the meatballs from the air fryer.  Add them to a pan over medium-low heat.  Coat meatballs with buffalo sauce and stir cooking in pan for 5-minutes.  Serve.

Nutrition: Calories:  302, Total Fat:  12.4g, Carbs:  7.6g, Protein:  32.1g

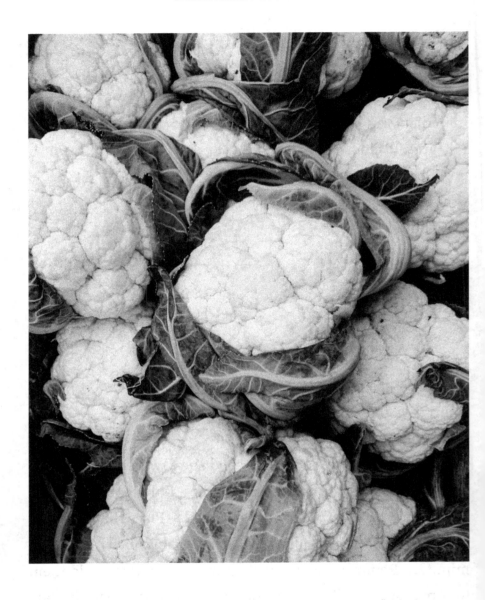

# Chapter 15. Bonus:

### 43. Harvest Pasta

Preparation Time: 35 Minutes

Servings:6

Ingredients

Kalamata olives – 1/3 cup (pitted)

Garlic – 2 cloves (minced)

White sugar – 1 tablespoon or more to taste

Dried oregano – 1 teaspoon

Vegetarian burger crumbs – ¾ cup

Diced tomatoes – 2 (14.5 ounce) cans

Bottled roasted red peppers – 1/3 cup (chopped)

Balsamic vinegar – 1 ½ tablespoons

Olive oil – 2 tablespoons

Black pepper to taste

Penne pasta – 1 pound

Instructions:

In a large saucepan, stir the olives, garlic, sugar, oregano, tomatoes, red pepper, vinegar. Bring this to simmer for about 20 to 30 minutes over medium high-heat before reducing to medium-low and let simmer until the sauce starts to thicken.

In a large pot, pour lightly salted water and boil over high heat. Once the water is boiling, put in the penne pasta and leave to boil.

Cook the pasta uncovered for about 11 minutes and remember to stir occasionally until the pasta is al-dente. After this drain.

Once the tomato sauce is done, pour it into the blender no more than halfway full. Hold down the lid and carefully start the blender using a few pulses to get the sauce moving before leaving it on to puree. Afterwards, puree until the mixture is smooth, then return to the pot.

Stir in the burger crumbles and simmer until it is hot. Then pour the finished sauce over the penne pasta to serve.

Nutritional facts:

Calories: 392; Fat: 8.8 g; Cholesterol: 0 mg; Carbohydrates: 64.9 g; Protein: 13.4 g; Iron: 6 mg; Calcium: 72 mg; Potassium: 345 mg.

Tips

You can also use a stick blender to puree the sauce in the pot until it is smooth.

## 44. Pollo Mediterranean

Preparation Time: 35 Minutes

Servings: 4

Ingredients

Olive oil – 2 tablespoons

Garlic – 3 cloves (minced)

Ground black pepper – ½ teaspoon

Sun-dried tomatoes packed in oi – ¼ cup (chopped and drained)

Dry white wine – ½ cup

Chicken tenders – 12 (sliced into strips)

Salt – ½ teaspoon

Italian seasoning – 1 tablespoon

Green olives – 2 tablespoons (sliced)

Fresh parsley – 2 tablespoons (chopped)

Sour cream – ½ cup

Salt – ½ teaspoon

Milk – 1 cup

Cornstarch – 1 ½ teaspoons

Water – ¼ cup

Instructions

In a skillet and over medium heat, heat olive oil. Place chicken and garlic in the pan. Season with pepper, Italian seasoning and ½ teaspoon of salt.

Stir in the olives, wine, parsley, tomatoes and olives then reduce heat to a low and continue cooking until the chicken is no longer pink at the center. Remove and place chicken on a late with the sauce still in the pan. Stir into the remaining sauce ½ teaspoon of sauce.

In a small bowl, whisk cornstarch and water together. Increase heat to the medium and whisk in the cornstarch mixture. Continue stirring until the sauce has thickened. Serve the sauce with chicken.

Nutritional fact:

Calories: 392; Fat: 19.7 g; Cholesterol: 111 mg; Carbohydrates: 9.2 g; Protein: 38 g; Calcium: 157 mg; Potassium: 590 mg.

Tips

You can use artichoke in the cooking.

## 45.   Pasta Fagioli Soup

Preparation Time: 75 Minutes

Servings: 8

Ingredients:

Water – 3 cups

Crisp cooked bacon – 8 slices (crumbled)

Dried parsley- 1 tablespoon

Garlic – 1 tablespoon (minced)

Garlic powder – 1 teaspoon

Ground black pepper – ½ teaspoon

Salt- 1 ½ teaspoon

Dried basil – ½ teaspoon

Tomato sauce – 1 (8 ounce) can

Seashell pasta – ½ pound

Great Northern beans – 2 (14 ounce) cans (undrained)

Chicken broth – 2 (14.5 ounce) can

Diced tomatoes – 1 (29 ounce) can

Chopped spinach – 1(14 ounce) can (drained)

Instructions

Combine all the other ingredients apart from pasta in a large stock pot to cook and boil. Let simmer for about 40 minutes.

Add pasta and cook with the pot uncovered until the pasta is tender. This should take approximately 10 minutes.

Serve.

Nutrition

Calories: 288; Fat: 3.6 g; Cholesterol: 7 mg; carbohydrates: 48.5 g; Protein: 15.8 mg; Iron: 5 mg; Calcium: 100 mg; Potassium: 701 mg

Tip

You can substitute half of the canned ingredients for better nutritional outcomes.

## 46.   Pasta al Mediterraneo

Preparation Time: 27 Minutes

Servings: 6

Ingredients

Perciatelli pasta – 1 pound

Pine nuts – 3 tablespoons (lightly roasted)

Fresh parsley – 2 tablespoons (chopped)

Lemon – 1 (juiced)

Can tuna – 2 (5 ounce) package (drained)

Kalamata olives – 12 (pitted and sliced)

Garlic – 1 clove (crushed)

Fresh basil – 4 ounces (chopped)

Olive oil – 6 tablespoons

Feta cheese – 2 ounces (optional)

Instructions

Cook pasta in a large bowl of slightly salted water until al dente. Meanwhile, mix in a large bowl, olives, garlic, basil, tuna, pine nuts, parsley and crumbled feta cheese.

Drain the pasta. If the plan is to serve cold, then rinse the pasta with cold water until it is no longer hot. In a large bowl, place pasta together with lemon juice and olive oil. Stir into the pasta mixture, the tuna mixture.

Serve hot or cold.

Nutritional fact

Calories: 519; Fat: 22 g; Cholesterol: 21 mg; Sodium: 255 mg; Carbohydrates: 59.5 g; Protein: 24.2 g; Calcium: 122 mg; Potassium: 370 mg.

Tips.

If possible, use fresh lemon juice instead of bottled ones.

## 47.    Tomato Basil Penne Pasta

Preparation Time: 45 Minutes

Servings: 4

Ingredients

Basil oil – 1 tablespoon

Garlic – 3 cloves (minced)

Pepper jack cheese – 1 cup

Parmesan cheese – ¼ cup (grated)

Basil oil – 1 tablespoon

Grape tomatoes – 1 pint (halved)

Mozzarella cheese – 1cup (shredded)

Fresh basil – 1 tablespoon (minced)

Instructions

Over high heat, bring a large pot of water to boil. Cook pasta in the boiling water for about 11 minutes until al dente, then drain.

In a large skillet and over medium-high heat, heat the basil and olive oil. Cook garlic in oil until soft. Afterwards, add tomatoes, reduce the heat to a medium and leave to dimmer for 10 minutes.

Stir in the mozzarella, parmesan cheese and pepper jack. When the cheese begins to melt, mix in the cooked penne pasta. Season with fresh basil.

Nutritional fact Calories: 502; Fat: 24.8 g; Cholesterol: 58 mg; Sodium: 462 mg; Carbohydrates: 47.1 g; Protein: 24.1 g; Calcium: 474 mg; Potassium: 311 mg. Tip

If basil oil is unavailable, use 2 tablespoons of olive oil

## 48. Whole Wheat Pasta Toss

Preparation Time: 45 Minutes

Servings: 8

Ingredients

Olive oil – 1/3 cup

Marinated artichoke hearts – 1 (8 ounce) jar (drained)

Kalamata olives – ¼ cup (pitted and quartered)

Feta cheese – ½ cup (crumbled)

Whole wheat penne pasta – 1 (1 pound) package

Garlic – 4 large cloves (pressed)

Pickled red peppers – 7 (cut into strips)

Fresh spinach leaves – 2 cups

Instructions

Fill a large bowl with lightly salted water and bring to boil. Put in the penne and continue to boil. Cook the pasta uncovered, stirring occasionally for 8 minutes or until al dente, then drain. In a large non-stick skillet and over medium heat, heat olive oil, the cook and stir in garlic into the hot oil for about 30 seconds until it is fragrant, for about 5 minutes. Gently fold the spinach into the mixture and stir just until slightly wilted and dark green.

Remove the mixture from heat and stir in the penne pasta until it is thoroughly combined; lightly toss pasta mixture in with the feta steam, cover the skillet with a lid and let the vegetables and pasta steam for about 10 minutes before serving.

Nutritional fact

Calories: 367; Fat :14.7 g; Cholesterol: 8 mg; Sodium: 347 mg; Carbohydrates: 47.4 g; Protein: 12.9 g; Iron: 1 mg; Calcium: 60 mg; Potassium: 58 mg

## 49.    Quick Mediterranean Pasta

Preparation Time: 25 Minutes

Servings: 6

Ingredients

Breadcrumbs – ¼ cup

Dried basil – 1 teaspoon

Spaghetti – 8 ounces

Dried oregano – 1 teaspoon

Olive oil – 1 tablespoon

Instructions

Boil slightly salted water in a large pot, put spaghetti in it and cook until al dente. Rinse and cool with water, then drain well. Mix the breadcrumbs, basil, oregano and cooked pasta in a large bowl. Pour as much olive oil as you would like over the mixture and serve.

Nutritional facts

Calories: 178; Fat: 3.1 g; Cholesterol: 0 mg; Sodium: 35 mg; Carbohydrate: 31.4 g; Protein: 5.5 g; Iron: 2 mg; Calcium: 25 mg; Potassium: 104 mg.

Tips

You can always experiment with the recipe

## 50.   Mongolian Chicken

Cooking Time: 17 minutes

Servings:  4

Ingredients:

4 chicken breasts, boneless, skinless, chopped small pieces

1 yellow onion, thinly sliced

Olive oil for frying

1 Chili Paid, chopped

3 garlic cloves, minced

5 curry leaves

1 teaspoon ginger, grated

¾ cup evaporated milk

Marinade:

1 egg

1 tablespoon light soy sauce

Self-rising flour to coat

½ tablespoon cornstarch

Seasonings:

1 teaspoon liquid stevia

1 tablespoon chili sauce

½ teaspoon sea salt

Dash of black pepper

Directions:

Combine all of you marinade ingredients in a bowl and marinate the chicken with it for an hour.  Dredge the chicken in the self-rising flour and spray some oil over.  Cook in air fryer for 10-minutes at 390°Fahrenheit. Heat a wok and sauté the ginger, garlic, chili paid, curry leaves and onions for 2-minutes. Add the chicken and seasonings, stirring to combine well. Add your milk and cook until thickened. Serve hot!

Nutrition: Calories: 286, Total Fat: 11.3g, Carbs: 6.4g, Protein: 28g

# Conclusion

Thank you for choosing and reading this book. We hope it was useful and able to provide you with a thorough overview of the Mediterranean diet, its lifestyle, its dos and don'ts. We hope this book has helped you understand more about this diet and given you the tools to set off on further research, to learn about the background of this diet and the food pyramid it is based on. Please remember, however, not to undergo any significant lifestyle or dietary changes without consulting your GP as there may be contraindications to certain elements. If this isn't your case, the Mediterranean diet will surprise you with its beneficial effects on your health, including but not limited to improving the appearance of your skin, lowering your cholesterol levels, helping prevent the onset of type 2 diabetes... all this in addition to losing weight!

CPSIA information can be obtained
at www.ICGtesting.com
Printed in the USA
BVHW090147280621
610620BV00005B/134

9 781801 915465